THE
BABY
SHOWER
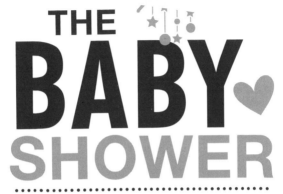

planning

GUIDE

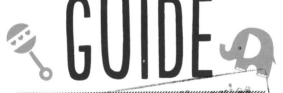

THE BABY SHOWER PLANNING GUIDE

Copyright © Summersdale Publishers Ltd, 2017

Text by Emily Kearns

Illustrations © Shutterstock

www.summersdale.com

Printed and bound in Malta

ISBN: 978-1-84953-748-3

Substantial discounts on bulk quantities of Summersdale books are available to corporations, professional associations and other organisations. For details contact general enquiries: telephone: +44 (0) 1243 771107, fax: +44 (0) 1243 786300 or email: enquiries@summersdale.com.

THE

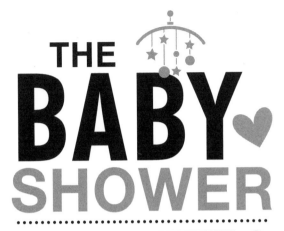

BABY

SHOWER

 planning

GUIDE

Emily Harper

summersdale

CONTENTS

INTRODUCTION

So you're planning a baby shower – welcome! If you've picked up this book it's likely you want to arrange something fun and a bit special that requires some thought and careful consideration. Just because the guest of honour is pregnant doesn't mean you can't plan something beyond tea, cake and gift exchanging. Why not celebrate the impending arrival but also make the most of her freedom while she's expecting?

In these pages you'll find suggestions for activities, which have been categorised into personality types to help you find something suitable for the mother-to-be. You'll also find a plethora of games – some sweet and some totally silly – as well as tons of crafting ideas, some for fun and others to create something special. There is also a section containing delicious mocktail and tasty snack recipes.

And don't forget – the theme doesn't always have to be baby-related. You could mix up the most obvious theme with something else that relates to the star guest's favourite hobbies or passions.

MAKING A PLAN

**FAIL TO PLAN,
PLAN TO FAIL.**

★ *Anonymous* ★

Will the mother-to-be want to get involved in eating ominous-looking brown foods out of disposable nappies and drinking mocktails out of baby bottles, or is she likely to turn her nose up at that sort of thing? Perhaps she would prefer something a little more refined – a picnic followed by a peaceful boat ride? Or maybe she'd enjoy being pampered at a spa and treated to afternoon tea. The chances are you know her well enough to be aware of her likes and dislikes. Put her first, but don't forget about the other guests. If a number of them suffer from motion sickness, for example, then a boat ride is not the way forward. Similarly, a host of hay fever sufferers might not enjoy a picnic in a delightful, but highly pollinated, grassy meadow. Whether it's a whole day's worth of activities you're planning or a simple tea party, take one step at a time and it'll all come together.

TO SURPRISE OR NOT?

The mother-to-be might love surprises – or she might loathe them. Some people like to have time to look forward to an event and find half the joy of it in the lead-up, whereas others really love being caught off guard with a celebration of what life has in store for them. Above all, make sure any surprises will go down well. Ask around her friends and family if you're not sure and then make a decision.

HOW TO CHOOSE A DATE

If the baby shower is not a surprise event, sit down with the mother-to-be and come up with a few potential dates. Do this as far in advance as possible – the more notice you give the guests the more likely most of them will be able to make it. And when it comes to arranging activities, you want to get in there before everything is booked up. You should also discuss with the mother-to-be or a relative how close to the due date to hold the shower. Leave it too late and the early arrival of the baby would scupper your plans. You might also find that the mother-to-be doesn't feel like doing very much the closer she gets to her due date, so opt for a date six to 12 weeks before.

Ask the guest of honour for a rough idea of what she'd like to do – would she like to go away for a weekend of pampering at a spa or stay closer to home? Perhaps she'd like to have a delicious lunch in an upmarket hotel, or maybe she'd prefer a DIY cream tea in the comfort of her own home.

If you are taking the surprise route, then perhaps ask her relatives or other close friends when they are available and consult with the mother-to-be's partner or someone close to her about when the person for whom you are throwing the party will be available. Let them know your ideas for the celebration and see if they are met with approval.

HOW TO SORT THE GUEST LIST

Talk to the mother-to-be about whom she would like to share her baby shower with. She might like the idea of a large crowd of people to have a day out with or she might prefer something more sedate with fewer guests. The number of guests will also affect the activities and games you can plan for the group, so it's good to get this all sorted as far in advance as possible.

Once you've got a clear idea of the kind of shower you are going to throw, gather the contact details of all those invited (the mother-to-be should be able to supply you with these, or if it's a surprise, the easiest way to contact the guests will probably be via Facebook or email) and send out a 'save the date' invitation. Introduce yourself, let them know they have been invited to a baby shower and add a sentence or two about what that might entail. Ask them to RSVP by a certain date – a week or two in the future should give them enough time – and chase them if they haven't replied by this date.

HOW TO CONTACT GUESTS

★ Email

★ Letter with perforated RSVP

★ Invitation card inside a decorated nappy

★ Postcard with picture of the mother-to-be

★ Social media group

★ WhatsApp group

★ Group text message

★ Cookie/marshmallow with date iced/printed on it

★ Pop-up card themed to the mother-to-be

★ Balloon with date printed on it

TIP *Rather than finding your inbox flooded with RSVPs, ask guests to fill in a quick and simple online poll to determine who is available when. Doodle.com is a good tool for this: simply follow the instructions, add the potential party dates and email the link to the guests. Once everyone has filled it in, you'll be able to see which dates are the most popular and when would be best to hold the party.*

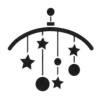

SAMPLE EMAIL TO GUESTS

Dear friends of ....,

Some of you know me, but for those who don't – hi! I'm [insert mother-to-be's name here]'s friend/sister/mother and I am organising a baby shower for her ahead of the exciting arrival in [insert month here].

We're looking at a few dates in [insert month(s) here] and it would be great if you could follow this link and let me know your availability [insert online poll link here].

I hope you can make it and look forward to hearing from you.

[insert your name here]

● ●

WHERE TO HOLD IT

● ●

Depending on what you plan to do in terms of activities and entertainment, you will need to think about where to hold the shower. If it's a surprise, perhaps you might want to hold it at a friend's or relative's house. If the mother-to-be has helped you plan it, she might just want everyone to come to her house. Or you might be planning to spend the evening in a restaurant or head out into the countryside for a day – there are plenty of ideas in these pages.

GIFTS

Guests will often want to bring gifts to a baby shower, but you don't want to find people doubling up. You could either set up a registry, similar to when people get married and set up a gift list, or find out what the mother-to-be still needs for the baby and set up an Amazon wishlist. Alternatively you could create and share a spreadsheet via Google Docs with a list of gifts and ask everyone to claim one, or add to it if they come up with a good idea. Make sure there is a mixture of gifts for mum as well as gifts for baby. You could also suggest clubbing together to buy something useful for the baby that the parents-to-be will have to buy anyway – to help ease the financial burden at what can be an expensive time.

BUDGET

If the guests earn wildly varying amounts, be sympathetic to that and keep the activities cheap – or hold a party in someone's house. The guests who earn the most can splash their cash on gifts for the baby if they want to make an extra contribution.

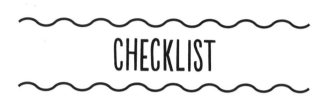

CHECKLIST

Before you do anything else, make a list of what needs to be done and in what order. Your list should look something like this:

★ Decide possible dates with mother-to-be (or her partner, if it is a surprise).

★ Gather list of guests' contact details from mother-to-be, her partner or family, or from social media.

★ Send out an email to guests to check they are available.

★ Sit down with the mother-to-be, or her partner or family, to discuss particulars.

★ Communicate with the guests about budget and loose plans so far and gather any deposits needed for accommodation or activities.

★ Do some more research with the above in mind.

★ Set a detailed budget if needed.

★ Book activities and gather any outstanding funds from guests.

★ Assign jobs to other guests if need be – people like to feel involved – but make sure they don't feel you're offloading too much of the work!

★ Send out an itinerary and accommodation details if needed, including requests for any props, etc. the guests need to bring with them.

★ Send an email to all the guests the week before the event, just to check everyone is prepared and has all the information they need.

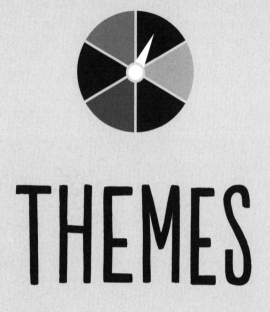

THEMES

THEME: SOPHISTICATED

SOPHISTICATION ISN'T WHAT YOU WEAR AND WHO YOU KNOW.

★ *Taylor Swift* ★

If the mother-to-be is a sophisticated sort, she might prefer something a bit more luxurious than a few once-frozen party snacks and a game of baby-themed charades. Surprise her with a spa day, where she has the chance to really unwind before life gets a bit more hectic, or take her out for a few mocktails in a classy setting. Take a look at the suggestions below and see how you get on.

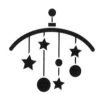

ACTIVITIES

AFTERNOON TEA AT A HOTEL

Many hotels and restaurants offer various afternoon tea packages – from the simple tea and cake, to mountains of scones with jam and lashings of cream, sweet treats and sandwiches, with perfectly prepared tea (ask ahead if they have caffeine-free, in case the mother-to-be loves a good brew but is avoiding caffeine) and sometimes even champagne cocktails (again, check they can provide non-alcoholic cocktails). This is a most pleasant and decadent way to spend an afternoon and provides a good opportunity for the mother-to-be to catch up with her friends and family before her new arrival.

A DAY AT THE RACES

Perhaps the mother-to-be has a penchant for a light flutter every now and again, and also any chance to wear a good hat. Bear in mind her stage of pregnancy – how far is she likely to want to walk and will she mind standing for long periods of time? If she's up for a day out, a trip to the races could be a good alternative for a baby shower celebration. Lots of companies offer race-day packages that include some refreshment and a meal. If you're working to a tighter budget, you could opt for a trip to a greyhound stadium (see page 55), posh hats optional.

MOCKTAILS AT A HOTEL ROOFTOP BAR

If the weather is on your side and you live in or close to a town or city, why not treat the mother-to-be to an evening of drinks at a swanky hotel rooftop bar. Alcohol may be off the menu, but do your research and find a place with a decent non-alcoholic cocktail offering. Reserve an area with a good view and ask the hotel nicely if you can bring a few decorations along – although, as this is the sophisticated chapter and the hotel is swanky, go for something a bit tasteful and possibly non-baby related (paper lanterns, fairy lights or some white fabric bunting should do the trick). Whether you've managed to hire a booth or a large table, as well as lots of chat, there are plenty of games you can play too (see page 84 for some ideas).

HACK: MOCKTAIL IT UP

To bring the budget down a little, why not create a selection of mocktails at home and serve them in some pretty glassware with all the accompanying straws and garnishes they deserve? Better still, does one of the guests happen to have a roof terrace, balcony or beautiful garden to host a drinks party? You could even string up some bunting and hang some fairy lights in the trees to make it a bit special. Make sure there's plenty of comfortable seating so everyone can relax and enjoy the ambience.

SPA DAY OUT OR WEEKEND AWAY

You might find what the mother-to-be would like more than anything is the chance to have a weekend away to relax before the baby arrives. Bear in mind that due to her condition she won't be able to enjoy the hot tub or sauna, so make sure the spa has suitable facilities and a nice pool so she won't feel left out if the other guests want to get stuck in. Do your research and find a spa that offers pregnancy massages or plenty of options including head, neck and shoulder, and hand and foot massages, as well as pedicures, manicures and facials. If she'd rather not be away for the whole weekend, find somewhere reasonably local that can accommodate you and make a day of it.

HACK:
DIY PAMPER PACKAGES

If you're working to a tight budget, why not bring the pampering in-house? Either hire a beautician or masseuse and get them to perform treatments at your or the mother-to-be's house (with a group the cost per person can be really reasonable for shorter treatments, like a 20-minute head and neck massage, for instance), or to bring the cost down further, perform treatments on each other. Don't worry about people who haven't met before having to perform full-body massages on each other – serious massage should not be attempted by the inexperienced, but there are plenty of alternatives. With some aromatherapy oils, a hand massage can be very pleasant; and it's easy enough to perform manicures on each other. Some oils are best avoided during pregnancy so do check first. You could also pick up a multipronged head massager and let the guests take it in turns using it on each other. Tell all guests to bring along a bathrobe and slippers and relax with a mocktail in hand.

GAMES

★ Famous mothers (see page 86)

★ Guess the size of the bump (see page 95)

★ What might the baby look like? (see page 100)

DECORATION IDEAS

★ Table confetti (either baby-themed or not)

★ Mocktail accessories

★ Paper lanterns with battery-operated tea lights

★ Tasteful fairy lights

★ White fabric bunting

THEME: OUTDOORS

IN ALL THINGS OF NATURE THERE IS SOMETHING OF THE MARVELLOUS.

★ *Aristotle* ★

Perhaps the mother-to-be likes to do nothing more in her spare time than hike up mountains, abseil over crags and kayak down local waterways. If this is the case, then the chances are she's had to cool it a little lately. She might really be missing the great outdoors and be grateful of a chance to get back to it, albeit in a slightly more relaxed capacity and with some toilets close by! She might not be all that bothered with adventure sports, but is simply a nature lover at heart – whatever the case, these suggestions should be a good fit.

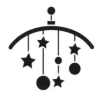

ACTIVITIES

VISIT A NATURE RESERVE

Check out your local Wildfowl & Wetlands Trust, RSPB Nature Reserve or beach and find out what activities they offer. Perhaps there are animals to observe or there might be a scenic trail to amble along. As long as it's not chucking it down with rain, snow or hail, this is a good option for the outdoor-loving mother-to-be. One thing's for sure, make sure there's a tearoom or a pub at the end of it and everyone will be happy. If there isn't a nature reserve nearby, it's likely there'll be some sort of pleasant green space, so seek one out and arrange a low-impact scenic walk... with a tearoom or a pub at the end of it.

PICNIC OR BARBECUE

Whether you opt for a picnic in a local park or a barbecue in someone's garden, this is a good option if you want to keep costs down and enjoy being outside. Make the picnic or barbecue a bit special and come up with some themed snacks and decorations – whether that theme is the baby or something the mother-to-be loves, such as animals, superheroes, Leonardo DiCaprio... These are also perfect settings for games that can get a bit messy (see page 84)! You could also organise a scavenger hunt to keep guests entertained. Again, come up with a theme to keep things interesting. Make sure you're well-equipped with a picnic rug or deckchair to keep the mother-to-be comfortable, and perhaps a parasol or umbrella to be prepared for any weather.

HACK:
GET EVERYONE INVOLVED

Trying to stick to a small budget can get a bit stressful, so if you're organising a picnic or a barbecue why not share the burden and ask all guests to each bring a dish or drinks. You could be extra organised about it and assign different foods and drinks to different guests. That way you'll end up with plenty to go round. You'll probably find that the other guests like being involved in the planning of the baby shower and will feel able to make their own suggestions. Set up a shared spreadsheet through Google Docs or similar to keep things in check. See page 122 for party snack recipes.

STAY IN A FOREST CABIN

Getting away for the weekend before the baby comes could be just what the mother-to-be is after and for the woman who loves the outdoors, relaxing in a forest cabin could be just the thing. Surrounded by woodland and countryside, with a plethora of walking trails, scenery and outdoor pursuits, there will be plenty to occupy the guests in the daytime, if they want it – the other alternative is to simply relax and watch the world go by. When evening comes guests can sit around a big campfire, play games, eat toasted marshmallows and drink hot chocolate. String up some pine cones and plenty of battery-operated fairy lights around the cabin to create a magical feel.

CANAL BOAT TRIP

Whether the nearest body of water is the sea, a river, canal or lake, there are plenty of options for a boat ride – and you could combine this with games and a picnic too. However, you might find the calmest waters to be found on a canal. And the mother-to-be may well love this idea, with someone else opening all of the locks while she puts her feet up and enjoys the company and scenery.

HEAD TO THE LIDO

If it's summer and your mother-to-be is a fan of swimming, why not head to the nearest open-air swimming pool for an afternoon of swimming and picnicking. (Be sure to take a break from swimming while you let your food go down.) As long as the weather is on your side, you can while away the whole day dipping in and out of the pool and, depending on the surrounding space, playing games and enjoying a barbecue or picnic. If there's enough room at your chosen spot, take along a croquet or badminton set – or both – and host a tournament.

HACK:
EARTH MOTHER PARTY

Keep costs down by throwing a baby shower at someone's house. If the mother-to-be is especially fond of environmental issues and doing her bit to save the planet, you could think about theming the shower around this. Organise a crafting session geared around upcycling and create something useful from things you might otherwise throw away or recycle. For example, you could create vases from old jars or pots and decorate them with ribbons, twine or paint. Be mindful about your party food and drink choices – if the mother-to-be is a sucker for a smoothie, create some delicious options and give them names related to the occasion, if you so wish (how about Green Goddess, Summer Sass, Berry Mama?). Use your imagination and dig through the recycling to create some colourful decorations to brighten up the place.

GAMES

★ Croquet, badminton or table tennis, if you have the kit

★ Scavenger hunt

★ Bobbing for bottles (see page 87)

★ Baby bottle bowling (see page 102)

DECORATION IDEAS

★ Pine cones, acorns and conkers on strings

★ Baby-themed piñata, perhaps in the shape of a baby bottle or a pram (preferably not a baby!)

★ Bunting and fairy lights

THEME:
CREATIVE

YOU CAN'T USE UP CREATIVITY. THE MORE YOU USE THE MORE YOU HAVE.

★ *Maya Angelou* ★

If the mother-to-be is a creative type, perhaps she would be up for learning a new skill or spending an afternoon crafting. You could plump for something a bit different and try a chocolate- or soap-making workshop. Whatever you go for, be aware of the other guests' skills and choose an activity the novice can master.

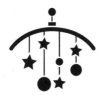

ACTIVITIES

CHOCOLATE-MAKING WORKSHOP

A chocolate-making workshop is perfect for creative or foodie types who don't mind getting their hands dirty – and the best thing about this activity is you get to eat the end product. Under expert tuition, learn how to make a variety of chocolate treats, and perhaps secretly craft chocolate letters to spell out 'it's a girl' or 'it's a boy' to present to the mother-to-be at the end of the day. You can assign a letter or letters to each guest to make as they go. Lots of events companies offer workshops like this, so it's highly likely you'll be able to find something in your local area.

HACK: CRAFTING

There are plenty of crafting activities you can organise on a small budget and you could even combine entertaining guests with creating a keepsake for the mother-to-be (see page 75). Arrange a crafting afternoon at your house (or the mother-to-be's or a relative's house if they have more space) and bring in the supplies. Think about creating jewellery, cosmetics, art and keepsakes. What are the mother-to-be's passions or hobbies? Have a think and come up with something geared towards her interests, and something she'll want to keep afterwards.

SOAP-MAKING WORKSHOP

For something a bit different, book a soap-making workshop and entertain the guests while you all make something unique and useful. With experts to guide you in making a batch of natural, handmade, personalised soap, you'll not only learn the basics of soap-making but also how to tailor it to your personal taste. You usually get to keep the whole batch and could package it nicely with tissue paper and ribbon, and give it to friends and family. Both a fun and informative experience, you can often find workshops that make a day of it and also include food and drink.

FANCY DRESS PARTY

If the mother-to-be has a penchant for dressing up you could organise a fancy dress party themed around something she loves. Perhaps she is really into superheroes or 1950s fashion, rock music or boy bands, gardening or pro-wrestling, baking or gaming. Whatever her passion, tailor the theme to it and get decorations to match. Or you could be adventurous and ask everyone to make their own outfit from things they have lying around the house. Offer a prize for the best effort.

· ·

GAMES

· ·

★ Pin the sperm on the egg (see page 96)

★ What might the baby look like? (see page 100)

★ Baby songs or films (see page 101)

DECORATION IDEAS

★ Homemade bunting or *papel picado* (Mexican tissue paper cut-out bunting-style flags)

★ Themed decorations for fancy dress party

★ Hanging paper pom-poms or lanterns

THEME: CULTURED

CULTURE IS THE WIDENING OF THE MIND AND SPIRIT.

★ *Jawaharlal Nehru* ★

If the mother-to-be likes nothing more than a weekend city break, a trip to the theatre, art galleries or museums, or curling up with a good book, then theme the baby shower around these activities. Perhaps she would relish a weekend away before the baby comes – head to a culture centre and soak it all up. Alternatively you could write your own quiz, tailored to her life and loves, or throw a literary-themed party.

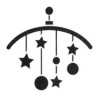

ACTIVITIES

THEMED TEA PARTY

Host a tea party with all the trimmings – cake, scones with jam and cream, towers of triangular sandwiches and gallons of tea (and caffeine-free alternatives) – and theme it around one of the mother-to-be's favourite books or TV programmes. Perhaps she loves Jane Austen novels or is partial to *Downton Abbey*. Encourage guests to dress up and let the mother-to-be realise her Lady Mary fantasies!

QUIZZES

Is the mother-to-be a quiz fiend? Or an avid watcher of *University Challenge* or *Mastermind*? Home-made quizzes could be just the ticket to kick off her baby shower festivities. Go for a mixture of rounds – history, geography, general knowledge, dates, food and drink, events and sport are just a few ideas. If you like you could add a few extra rounds in there themed towards babies – perhaps a 'name the celebrity baby' picture round or get guests to guess the celebrity you're describing from one fact about them and their date of birth. Another twist on the picture round could be gathering pictures of all the guests when they were infants and asking everyone to guess who is who (see page 85). Print out some quiz sheets and act as quizmaster.

THEATRE TRIP

To satisfy the culture vultures, why not check out your local theatre listings and see if there are any performances suited to the occasion. If your mother-to-be is a musicals enthusiast and you live close enough, you could head to London for the day where there are numerous shows to choose from. To keep costs down you could do some research into the many discount theatre ticket websites out there. (Just make sure the website you use is legitimate.) Make a day of it in the Big Smoke and combine with an afternoon tea-style experience or a bit of pampering for the mother-to-be. Just remember to not make the day too strenuous as the mother-to-be may tire sooner than others.

HACK: PUT ON A PLAY

If you don't have the budget for theatre tickets, you could always put on a play yourself. This might take a bit of planning and liaising with the other guests, but it could be rather fun and is definitely something the mother-to-be will not forget in a hurry! Write the play yourself and tailor it towards the guest of honour and the fact she is about to become a mother (or if she is already a mother, then just theme it around her life). If your creative juices aren't flowing, pick a well-known story, or perhaps her favourite soap opera, and adapt it – make it funny, pepper it with personal jokes and change character names so everyone plays a part. You could always perform and film it ahead of the day and host a screening on the day of the shower. Alternatively, if that all sounds like too much effort, why not ask guests to write a poem or song about the mother-to-be and either perform it for her on the day or you could all get together to create a pop video beforehand and host a screening at the shower.

WEEKEND OF CULTURE

A weekend away could be just what the mother-to-be needs before the baby is born. Why not organise a city break that combines culture with relaxation? Bath is not only brimming with culture – think Jane Austen and the Romans – but also offers the ultimate in relaxation at the Thermae Bath Spa, the country's only natural thermal spa. Bath is not a huge place so everything is quite close together. Alternatively, make a beeline for Liverpool or Manchester, where galleries and cultural activities abound. Stay in a comfortable hotel or a city apartment, booked through Airbnb or similar, where you can cook for each other, have the space to play games and can relax in pleasant surroundings.

GAMES

★ Name that children's book (see page 98)

★ Fill in the blanks (see page 99)

★ Baby-related anagrams (see page 99)

DECORATION IDEAS

★ Paper bunting featuring lines from nursery rhymes or famous literary quotes

★ Decorations featuring extracts from famous children's books

★ Paper table ornaments featuring trivia

★ Items themed to her favourite book or TV series as table decorations

THEME: OUTGOING

NEVER, EVER UNDERESTIMATE THE IMPORTANCE OF HAVING FUN.

★ *Randy Pausch* ★

If the mother-to-be is something of a party animal, she might have had to rein it in a little recently. Inject some fun back into things with a few rounds of karaoke or a trip to the dogs for a light flutter. Play some raucous party games and show her a good time.

ACTIVITIES

A TRIP TO THE DOGS

If your mother-to-be has a penchant for a scratch card or two or buys lottery tickets every week, organise a trip to the local greyhound stadium and let her try her luck on a few races. Most stadiums offer very reasonable packages that include pie and chips, a drink and a couple of bets. You can tease the mother-to-be and tell her that if your dog wins, she'll have to name her child after it. A light flutter is all fun and games as long as no one raises the stakes TOO high. Perhaps set a budget beforehand!

KARAOKE

Who says you need to drink alcohol to get involved in karaoke? There are plenty of folk who will happily burst into song at any given opportunity. Perhaps your mother-to-be is one of them! Many towns and cities now offer private karaoke booths where you can sit in a padded room away from the crowds and sing to each other, usually with the added help of a box of silly stuff like wigs and inflatable guitars. If the guest of honour isn't currently feeling like the night owl she once was, don't worry, just book an early slot.

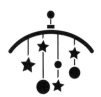

HACK: DIY KARAOKE

If you'd rather keep things cheap, there aren't any private karaoke booths nearby or you'd rather organise an activity in the day time, then simply bring the karaoke in-house. Ask around the guests to see if anyone has a suitable video game (SingStar and Guitar Hero are perennial favourites) and the respective games console that they can bring with them. Set it all up round someone's house and sing your hearts out. Chuck everyone's name in a hat and pull them out two at a time so they can belt out duets together, whatever the time of day.

PERFUME-MAKING WORKSHOP

With experts on hand to guide you in creating a perfume geared towards your favourite scents, this is a great activity for any mother-to-be who has a perfume collection to rival the best of them. Guests will smell their way through a plethora of ingredients and learn how best to blend them to make the perfect fragrance to suit them. With access to all the professional materials, you can trial-and-error your way through an afternoon until you come up with a winning scent.

CRANIUM TOURNAMENT

The board game for the louder party guest, Cranium requires players to do impressions, hum and sing. You can play in teams so this game works for any number of players, depending on how many guests you have to entertain. Ask around the guests to see who has a copy of the game and if you're out of luck just invent your own version of it with simpler rules. Come up with lists of songs and TV theme tunes for teams to hum to each other, tricky words to spell, strange words to define, items to draw or be moulded out of Play-Doh, while the other members of the team try to guess the answer. If this all sounds too complicated, dig out your copy of Pictionary or play a loud game of charades.

GAMES

★ *X Factor*-style karaoke tournament

★ Buggy racing (see page 92)

★ Pregnant Twister (see page 100)

★ Aim for the potty (see page 104)

DECORATION IDEAS

★ Animal-print-themed decorations

★ Homemade bunting featuring favourite musicians

★ Brightly coloured streamers

★ Entertaining photos of the mother-to-be

THEME: INTROVERT

QUIET PEOPLE HAVE THE LOUDEST MINDS.

★ *Stephen Hawking* ★

Perhaps the mother-to-be would rather stay closer to home – her living room to be exact – and have a pyjama party accompanied by her favourite films or TV shows, with themed decorations and games. Or maybe she's a nature lover and would enjoy a non-strenuous ramble through local greenery, away from the crowds. She might be the creative type, in which case there are options galore – think pottery painting, candle-making or cupcake decorating.

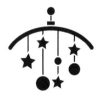

ACTIVITIES

FLASH FICTION WRITING

Do you have a bunch of budding writers in the house? Or a mother-to-be who is herself something of a scribe or has an interest in it? Send all the guests off to put pen to paper for 5–10 minutes only and come up with a piece of fiction of less than 100 words that stars the mother-to-be as a central character. (Perhaps the mother-to-be can write a piece of fiction about what she imagines her life to be like in six months' time.) When the time is up, all guests should reconvene and take it in turns to read out their creations. The funnier the better! The best thing about this activity is that it is 100 per cent free and can be loads of fun. If you'd rather skip the fiction, opt for a true story involving the writer and the mother-to-be – again, the funnier the better and encourage everyone to be as descriptive as possible.

A DAY IN THE COUNTRYSIDE

Perhaps your mother-to-be likes long country walks with warm fires at the end of them, or rambling through nature, spotting wildlife and foraging, all the while hunting down the best vistas around. As long as it's relatively dry, an afternoon of pleasant ambling through woodland – or a nature reserve or national park – with her nearest and dearest could be just what she wants from a baby shower celebration. If the weather is fine, combine it with a picnic; if it's a little chilly, make sure there's a pub nearby with a roaring fire so everyone can warm up before heading home.

CINEMA TRIP

If the mother-to-be is something of a film buff she might like a trip to the cinema before the baby comes along and visits to the big screen potentially fall off for a while. Local independent cinemas sometimes offer a more luxurious experience than the mainstream – do some research and see if there's one nearby where the mother-to-be can enjoy a film from the comfort of a plush sofa, while sipping on hot chocolate. These cinemas often have cafe/bar/restaurant spaces, so it could all be tied in with the cinema experience. Round off the day with a film quiz and gear it towards actors or directors as babies or young children. (See page 49.)

HACK: FILM PARTY

If you'd rather keep costs down and watch films from the comfort of a sofa, why not host a movie pyjama party? Perhaps she has a favourite trilogy, director or actor – depending on your guests' stamina you could screen two or three films back to back with a game played in between each. If people don't want a late night, start early and draw the curtains. String up decorations themed around the films that will be screened, serve mocktails and snacks that tie in with them too, and ask guests to bring extra cushions with them so everyone can get comfortable.

AN AFTERNOON OF CREATIVITY

If the mother-to-be is a fan of making things, you could book a creative workshop. Pottery-painting studios can be found all over the country, if you think this is something that she would enjoy. Alternatively you could opt for something a bit different like candle-making – check out what is available locally. If the guest of honour is a *Great British Bake Off* superfan then a cupcake-decorating class could be a good shout. And the best thing about that is you all get to gorge on your creations afterwards.

BOX-SET MARATHON

Perhaps the mother-to-be is a *Friends* obsessive, or adores *Sherlock*, *The X-Files* or *Buffy the Vampire Slayer*. Whatever her televisual kryptonite, select the best five or six episodes (or if you have the time and depending on the length of the episodes, go the whole hog and do a top ten, starting with ten and working down to the best/the mother-to-be's favourite). As you would with the film party, gear the accompanying games and decorations around the TV series and you could even introduce props if your guest of honour is *really* into this show. Pyjamas and extra cushions, popcorn and fizzy drinks optional.

GAMES

★ Name that baby animal (see page 90)

★ Guess the animal's gestation period (see page 91)

★ The price is right (see page 94)

DECORATION IDEAS

★ Pine cones, acorns and conkers on strings

★ Popcorn on strings, and film and TV show stills

THEME: QUIRKY

**IF THEY SAY I'M QUIRKY,
I'M QUIRKY. IT'S BETTER
THAN BEING BORING.**

★ *Zooey Deschanel* ★

For the more out there mother-to-be, let your imagination run wild. The chances are she will love it if you come up with something a bit different, so don't be afraid to be bold. If you think she'd like to be whisked away for the weekend, make sure the accommodation and activities are weird and wonderful; if she'd rather stay at home, bring the party to her and arrange vintage makeovers and a tea party themed to her favourite era.

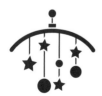

ACTIVITIES

VINTAGE MAKEOVER AND TEA PARTY

There are lots of companies that will provide everything you need to host a vintage tea party, complete with vintage crockery, waitresses, cream tea, a glass of bubbly and special gifts for the mother-to-be. There's also the option to add vintage make-up or hair styling packages, with several decades' worth of styles to choose from. Who says one can't get dolled up in glamorous gear to sit around drinking tea? These packages are usually geared towards hen parties but there's no reason why they can't be adapted for a baby shower. Call ahead and discuss options with the experts – they'll be able to make some suggestions and might even come up with some vintage-inspired mocktails for the occasion.

WEIRD AND WONDERFUL WEEKEND AWAY

If you think the mother-to-be would relish a weekend away before the baby arrives, why not plan something a bit special and opt for some unusual accommodation. There are so many options – from refurbished train carriages, to luxury yurts, beautiful tree houses, Hobbit-style pods, medieval castles, houseboats, lighthouses, sea forts, windmills and more. Pack up and head off for a memorable weekend full of relaxation and quality time with each other.

HAND AND FOOT CASTS

For something a bit different, you could arrange to take a cast of the mother-to-be's hand and foot and, as a gift, either present her with a kit to make a cast of the baby's hands and feet when it arrives, or a voucher for a professional to do it. The mother-to-be's casts could be made either at home with a kit or at a studio – if the latter, why not combine it with a trip to a nearby restaurant/tearoom?

SENSORY PARTY

Theme the baby shower around games that involve the senses – separate the guests into two teams and let the teams take it in turns to be blindfolded and guess what certain things are. You can ask guests to taste certain foods – baby food is always a favourite at baby showers – smell certain foods, drinks or perhaps even baby products such as nappy rash cream or baby wipes – use your imagination! You could also get the mother-to-be to feel certain objects she will be using in the not too distant future when the baby comes along and get her to guess what each one is. Alternatively the gift-giving could be done blindfolded and the mother-to-be has to guess what each item she unwraps actually is.

HACK: GAMING

If the mother-to-be is a keen gamer, why not hold a tournament or an afternoon/evening of gaming for everyone to enjoy. Does one of the guests own a Wii or an Xbox Kinect? Can you lay your hands on some games that particularly reflect the mother-to-be's interests or loves? If you can't find anyone to lend, second-hand game/DVD shops often sell these at reasonable prices and you can sell the games back to the shop afterwards if you don't want to keep them. Set it all up in the biggest living room to be found among you, push the sofas to the edges of the room and load up the side tables with snacks and party food, and let the games begin.

GAMES

★ Change that nappy – blindfolded (see page 103)

★ Guess the poo (see page 89)

★ Guess the baby food (see page 88)

DECORATION IDEAS

★ Bunting made from ultrasound pictures of baby

★ Vintage-style bunting and coloured fairy lights

★ Sensory decorations, made to be touched – make these out of bubble wrap, super-soft fabric, fake fur or noisy, scrunchy cellophane

THINGS TO MAKE AND DO

KEEPSAKES FOR THE MOTHER-TO-BE

THE BEST GIFTS COME FROM THE HEART, NOT THE STORE.

★ *Sarah Dessen* ★

BABY BIB DECORATING

Buy as many plain white cotton bibs as you have guests and plenty of fabric pens in a variety of colours. Ask guests to take a bib and some pens each and let their creative juices run wild. Tell them to be funny, imaginative or just plain silly. The bibs will raise a smile when the mother-to-be is cleaning bits of food off the little one and she'll remember her friends and the celebration fondly.

BABYGRO DECORATING

Similarly to the bib decorating, if you have a slightly bigger budget (if you feel comfortable, you could ask the guests to chip in a little for this) you could buy as many plain white Babygros as you have guests, along with fabric pens and maybe even some shapes or stencils to draw around – think animals, space, nature or simple shapes. Ask guests to decorate the all-in-ones however they desire. Not only will these please the mother-to-be when she is dressing the new baby, but they will no doubt be extremely useful when the baby needs to be changed several times a day!

LETTER WRITING

Simple and cheap, yet an invaluable keepsake for the mother-to-be. All you need for this is a stack of envelopes and paper, along with pens (coloured felt tips if you like for decoration) and perhaps some stickers, etc. Ask each guest to write a letter to the mother-to-be for her to read in hospital or when she gets back home after the birth, and decorate it however they would like. She will be tired and no doubt hugely appreciate the letters of love, support, perhaps humour – whatever you think suits.

NAPPY DECORATING

Another keepsake for the mother-to-be that doesn't cost the earth, but will be hugely appreciated. Buy a pack of nappies for newborns and some fabric pens or permanent markers. Test the pens out on the nappies you have bought first to make sure they write well on the material. Ask guests to decorate a few nappies each with jokes, short messages, patterns or drawings. Be as creative or amusing as you like – these are entirely for the mother-to-be's benefit and will lift her spirits when she's changing the little one's nappy at 3 a.m. after poomageddon.

ADVICE BOOK

If the mother-to-be's friends have already become parents, great, but if not do not worry, you can still create an advice book. Ask guests to each bring a photo of themselves – maybe even with the mother-to-be – or even better get hold of a Polaroid-style camera and take the photos on the day. Assign a page to each guest, affix the photo and ask them to relay a piece of advice to help the mother-to-be in the coming months. Don't worry if you have no experience of being a parent yourself; you may still have some good ideas or you could scour the internet for some amusing life hacks and make a little list for your friend.

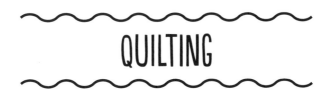

QUILTING

This one takes a bit of preparation and requires a good quilter or a sewing party to put it all together at the end, but the result will be a lovely keepsake for the mother-to-be and will last for a long time. Gather together some large squares of fabric – the size will depend on how many guests you are expecting as the number of squares you end up with will need to be big enough to make a good sized quilt. Only a few squares? No problem – just make a baby-sized quilt. You'll need sewing equipment, sequins, fabric pens and ribbons, etc. – whatever you think people are likely to want to use to decorate their square. Gather them all up at the end and hand over to your crafty friend to create the finished article, or put them together... together.

PRAM BLANKET

Ask guests to knit or crochet a square (or multiple squares if they can – the more the merrier!) ahead of the shower. Supply them with the measurements and needle size so they all turn out roughly the same size. You can also ask family members and friends of the mother-to-be who live abroad or can't make it on the day to join in with this gift. There are no rules when it comes to colour – this will make for a characterful blanket like no other. Ask the most creative of your group to stitch all the squares together – you can either do this before the shower or, if easier, ask guests to bring the squares to the shower and show the mother-to-be what you have all created. Tell her they will all come together to make a blanket for the new arrival and present it to her once the baby arrives.

BOX OF SURPRISES

Create a box of surprises for your mother-to-be to open when she gets home from the hospital. This could include luxury bath items, some mini-bottles of wine, chocolates, massage oils and, depending on your budget, maybe even a lovely new fluffy dressing gown, slippers or pyjamas. Include notes from the guests or all sign a big card to slip into the box with the gifts.

GAMES

**LIFE IS MORE FUN IF
YOU PLAY GAMES.**

★ *Roald Dahl* ★

NAME THAT BABY

Ask each guest to bring a photo of themselves as a baby (if you're throwing a surprise shower, ask a relative of the mother-to-be to bring a photo of her). Number them all and ask the guests to write down which guest they think each baby photo belongs to. Gather all the answer sheets and award a prize to the guest who scores the most points.

FAMOUS MOTHERS

Prepare by writing out the names of famous mothers on separate sheets of paper. Ideas for famous mothers (real or fictional) could be: Mother Goose, Mrs Bennet, Beyoncé, Angelina Jolie, Princess Diana, etc. As each guest arrives, pin one of the pieces of paper to their back. As the baby shower progresses, guests should ask each other yes or no questions about the name and once they have guessed correctly they may remove the name from their back. This is an especially good ice-breaker if many of the guests haven't met before.

BOBBING FOR BOTTLES

Like bobbing for apples at Halloween parties, tie up your hair, place your hands behind your back and 'bob' for the plastic 'nipple' tops of baby bottles bobbing in the water of a washing-up bowl. All the memories of Brownie camp will come flooding back. Set a time limit and see who can grab the most bottle tops in their teeth in the space of a minute.

GUESS THE BABY FOOD

Classic baby shower game this one – simply head to the baby food aisle in the supermarket and do your worst. There are so many different ones on offer these days that you'll be able to pick up an interesting selection for the guests to try. Place the puréed baby foods into unmarked containers and encourage guests to taste and then write down any flavours they think they detect.

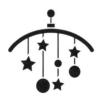

GUESS THE POO

This one isn't for everyone. It's really quite disgusting, but then some mothers-to-be, depending on the maturity level of their sense of humour, might find it totally hilarious. Take five to ten different chocolate bars and melt each one into a different nappy. Line them all up on a table and ask guests to guess the brand and type of chocolate bar. Use well-known ones so they have a chance of guessing correctly. And allow them a little taste if they're struggling – if they want to go anywhere near them that is.

NAME THAT BABY ANIMAL

A good one for animal lovers, or anyone really as who can resist cooing at baby animals... Print out some pictures of newborn baby animals when they don't quite look themselves yet. Try to find pictures that aren't too obvious, so it will encourage your guests to think about it and discuss it – another good ice-breaker. Divide guests into teams and offer a prize for whoever lands the most correct answers.

GUESS THE ANIMAL'S GESTATION PERIOD

Always a good one to get guests thinking and discussing, most likely casting their minds back to biology lessons many moons ago. This one takes a little preparation. Print out a list of animals and the length of their gestation period – this is your copy. Then delete the answers and print out a sheet for each guest or each team if you decide to group guests together. Once all the answers have been filled in, gather in the sheets and work out who has been victorious. Perhaps you could offer something animal-related as the prize – a soft toy in the form of a baby elephant perhaps? Elephants have one of the longest gestation periods at 20–21 months.

BUGGY RACING

If the guest list features many mothers, you might find there are a few babies at the shower. That could then mean there are several buggies – perfect for racing! No mothers or babies? Borrow a couple of buggies and set up an obstacle course. Pitch guests against each other in sets of two and hold a tournament-style competition so guests can battle it out for some sort of trophy that you will have lovingly handcrafted.

HOW MANY SWEETS IN THE BABY BOTTLE?

Fill a baby bottle with sweets (make sure you count them and take a note of the total somewhere) and place on a table with a sheet of paper and a pen. Draw a table on the piece of paper with room for the guest's name and their guess. As people mill around the party, ask them to write down their name and take a good guess at how may sweets they think are in the baby bottle. Wait until everyone has had a turn and then announce the winner. Whoever comes closest gets to keep the baby bottle and contents.

THE PRICE IS RIGHT

An easy one for mothers, perhaps, but an eye-opener for non-mothers. Take a decent selection of baby products available in a supermarket, for ease, things like baby shampoo, nappies, baby food, formula milk, baby bottle, baby wipes, talcum powder, rusks, etc. Use your imagination, or let the supermarket aisle guide you. If you don't want to shell out for these things and don't have a child yourself, you can always borrow them from another guest. Make some large price tags with the correct prices on and mix them up. Set all items on a table, along with the mixed-up price tags and ask the guests to assign a price to each item.

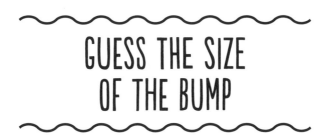

GUESS THE SIZE OF THE BUMP

As soon as the mother-to-be arrives, whisk her off to one side and measure the size of her bump. Make a note of this somewhere safe for later. When the time comes, ask guests to submit their guesses and write them down on a sheet of paper along with their name. Gather all the guesses together and work out who has come closest. Make sure you have a prize on hand to offer to the victor.

PIN THE SPERM ON THE EGG

Fairly self-explanatory this one – although it will take a little preparation on your part. Flex your best creative muscles and draw a lovely big egg on a large piece of card. Give it an outside and a much smaller centre, which is what guests will aim for. Borrow an artist's easel (or perhaps you have one yourself; after all, you just used your artistic talents to draw a big egg) to rest it on and fashion several sperms from some more cardboard. Attach some sticky fixer to the back and arm each guest with their own sperm. Guests should be blindfolded a few metres away from the easel and pointed in the right direction, where they then attach their sperm to the egg, as close to the centre as possible. Remove blindfold and let hilarity ensue.

DON'T SAY 'BABY'

Now here's a challenge. On arrival, hand out some pegs to the party guests – say, two or three each, depending on how many you have. Instruct guests as to the rules of the game – they may not, under any circumstances, say the word 'baby'. This is a tough one! If anyone slips up they must hand one of the pegs over to whoever was closest when they said the forbidden word. Once all your pegs are gone you don't have to play any more and can speak as freely as you like – this will also make it harder for the players still in the game. Whoever has the most pegs at the end of the game wins.

NAME THAT CHILDREN'S BOOK

Compile a list of best-known lines from children's books – these can be current, especially if your guests have children, but if there are no other mothers present you might want to lean heavily towards books from the era of their childhood. Print out a copy of the lines for each guest and ask them to name the book and, for an extra point, the author too. Present whoever gets the most correct answers with a prize, perhaps one of the books featured in the game.

FILL IN THE BLANKS

Take some well-known nursery rhymes and print them out with some words omitted. Ask guests to work in teams to fill in the blanks to complete the verse. To make this more challenging or possibly much more amusing, go for some obscure nursery rhymes and omit words that could potentially be replaced with something rather rude – and see what your guests come up with!

BABY-RELATED ANAGRAMS

There are lots of anagram generators on the internet, so pick one and come up with some good anagrams for baby or pregnancy-related words. Print out sheets for the guests featuring the scrambled words and a place for their answer. Offer a prize for the best word unscrambler.

PREGNANT TWISTER

For this one all you'll need is the board game Twister and a pack of balloons. Blow up the balloons, ask each guest (apart from the mother-to-be and anyone else who's pregnant) to place one under their shirt if they can, and play Twister.

WHAT MIGHT THE BABY LOOK LIKE?

Print out large versions of the mother-to-be, father-to-be, and relatives too, if you like, and cut them into strips widthways, so they look like slices of a Photofit. Make two sets so guests can work in teams and ask them to come up with what they think the baby will look like. Results are likely to be hilarious and possibly quite creepy.

BABY SONGS OR FILMS

Give each guest a sheet of paper and a pen. Choose either songs or films, depending on what you think the guests would most enjoy (or both!), set a timer for, say, two minutes, and ask the guests to write down as many titles as they can that feature the word 'baby'. Offer a prize for the longest list.

NAME THE BABY

Ask guests to write down their suggestions for first or middle names for the baby. Place all suggestions into a bowl/bag and ask the mother-to-be to read them out. Most are likely to be hilarious, but you never know… she might actually take a shine to some of them!

BABY BOTTLE BOWLING

This one is best played in the garden, or perhaps the kitchen if you have a particularly large one. Get hold of nine baby bottles and place a little sand or gravel into the base of each. Set them up in a triangle formation and get guests to take it in turns to bowl a tennis ball in their direction to see how many they can floor.

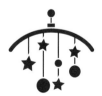

CHANGE THAT NAPPY – BLINDFOLDED

You'll need some dolls for this one – one will do if you want to time each participant, although it will be more fun to have a couple and let guests race each other. Set out a bottle of talcum powder and a pile of nappies next to the doll and ask guests, while blindfolded, to talc the baby's bottom and then put the nappy on. This might get a bit messy, so maybe put down some plastic sheeting or play outside!

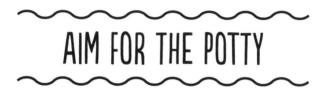

AIM FOR THE POTTY

Borrow some potties from friends who are parents, or improvise using buckets or large bowls. Depending on the amount of space and equipment you have, you may want to get guests to race against each other two at a time rather than all at once. Place the potties at the end of the room or garden and give each guest a blown-up balloon and ask them to put it under their shirt (the mother-to-be or any other pregnant guests don't need to do this bit). Then give everyone a 10p piece, ask them to hold it between their knees and get them to race to the potty and drop it in. Perhaps play in teams and see how many coins each team can accumulate.

MOCKTAIL RECIPES

LEARN HOW TO HAVE FUN WITHOUT ALCOHOL, TALK WITHOUT MOBILE PHONES, LOVE WITHOUT CONDITIONS, SMILE WITHOUT SELFIES.

★ *Anonymous* ★

You don't need booze to create delicious cocktails. Check out these takes on some classic serves. Offer a Virgin Mary or Strawberry 'Mimosa' at a brunch-style party, Mango Fizz or Pink Grapefruit Cooler at a picnic, or kick off the evening with some Sham-pagne or a Nojito. Make sure you have the right cocktail-making kit and glassware, as well as decorations and garnishes, to make these as authentic as possible. Each of the recipes below is for one serving.

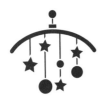

VIRGIN MARY

INGREDIENTS

200 ml tomato juice
1 tsp lemon juice
½ tsp Tabasco sauce
½ tsp Worcestershire sauce
   (vegetarian versions are available,
   but check ingredients to be sure)
A pinch of celery salt
A pinch of black pepper
Garnish of your choice (see recipe)

METHOD

Mix all of the ingredients well in a cocktail shaker if you have one, add some ice and serve in a tall glass. Garnish with a stick of celery, cucumber, basil leaves or, if you're feeling adventurous, a tall rasher of crispy, streaky bacon. Tip: If everyone is drinking Virgin Marys, make up jugs of it without the Tabasco (too spicy for some) and Worcestershire sauce (if non-vegetarian) and leave the bottles out for people to add it themselves.

ALCOHOL-FREE MIMOSA

INGREDIENTS

100 ml orange juice, smooth or with bits
100 ml ginger ale
¼ tsp grenadine or strawberry purée
Orange slices, to garnish

METHOD

Mix the orange juice and grenadine together and then add the ginger ale. Add strawberry purée instead of grenadine for a different twist on this mocktail.

NOJITO

INGREDIENTS

250 ml ginger ale, soda water or lemonade
1 tbsp fresh lime juice
1 tsp sugar
5 mint leaves
Crushed ice
Sprig of mint, to garnish (optional)

METHOD

Place the mint leaves, lime juice and sugar into a tall glass and muddle well. Add a handful or two of crushed ice and top with ginger ale, soda water or lemonade, depending on how sweet you want the end result to be. Give the whole lot a good stir and then top with more crushed ice if needed and a sprig of mint to garnish.

SHAM-PAGNE

INGREDIENTS

250 ml soda water
60 ml lime cordial
60 ml elderflower cordial
Fresh raspberry, to garnish

METHOD

Pour the lime cordial, elderflower cordial and soda water into a jug and give it a good stir. Pour into a champagne glass and add a raspberry to the drink to serve.

RASPBERRY—LIME COOLER

INGREDIENTS

125 ml soda water
4 tsp lime juice
8 raspberries
Ice cubes
Dash of grenadine
Fresh raspberry and mint leaves, to garnish (optional)

METHOD

Crush the raspberries in the bottom of a tall glass and add the lime juice. Give it a good stir. Add the ice and top with soda water. Give it another good stir with a straw and add a dash of grenadine to float in the drink. Garnish with raspberries and mint leaves as desired.

MANGO FIZZ

INGREDIENTS

125 ml ginger ale
25 ml sugar syrup
25 ml lime juice
25 ml mango purée
5 mint leaves
Crushed ice
Sprig of mint, to garnish (optional)

METHOD

Place the mint, sugar syrup, lime juice and mango purée in a tall glass and muddle gently. Add a handful or two of crushed ice, until the glass is two-thirds full, and fill the rest of the glass with ginger ale. Give the whole thing a good stir, add more crushed ice if needed and garnish with a sprig of mint.

PINEAPPLE PASSION

INGREDIENTS

60 ml pineapple juice
30 ml passion fruit juice
30 ml lemon juice
Dash of grenadine
Ice cubes
Pineapple wedge, to garnish (optional)

METHOD

Mix all ingredients together in a cocktail shaker, if you have one, and shake well with the ice. Strain into a Martini glass for some extra class. If you want to go the whole hog, add a cocktail umbrella and a pineapple wedge to the rim.

ORANGE AND LEMON FIZZ

INGREDIENTS

2 oranges, juiced
2 tsp lemon juice
2 tsp sugar syrup
Splash of sparkling water
Crushed ice
Sprig of mint and/or orange and lemon zest strips,
   to garnish (optional)

METHOD

Juice the two oranges and mix together with the lemon
juice and sugar syrup. Strain into a tall glass filled with
crushed ice and top it up with sparkling water. Add
some more crushed ice if desired and garnish with a
sprig of mint and/or orange and lemon zest strips.

PINK GRAPEFRUIT COOLER

INGREDIENTS

1 grapefruit, juiced
½ lemon, juiced
40 ml sugar syrup
Splash of soda water
A few mint leaves
Crushed ice
Slice of grapefruit or sprig of mint, to garnish (optional)

METHOD

Muddle the sugar syrup and mint in the bottom of a tall glass. Juice the grapefruit and lemon and add to the glass along with the ice. Top the lot with soda water and garnish with a sprig of mint and a slice of grapefruit if desired.

SHIRLEY TEMPLE

INGREDIENTS

200 ml ginger ale
Dash of grenadine
Maraschino cherry
Ice cubes

METHOD

Pour the ginger ale into a tall glass over ice. Add a dash of grenadine along with the maraschino cherry.

BLUEBERRY SMASH

INGREDIENTS

125 ml sparkling water
30 ml lemon juice
30 ml sugar syrup
8 blueberries
1 sprig of rosemary
Ice cubes
Blueberries and rosemary, to garnish (optional)

METHOD

Muddle the blueberries, rosemary and sugar syrup in a cocktail shaker. Add the lemon juice and ice and shake well. Strain into a tall glass over fresh ice. Top with sparkling water and garnish with more blueberries and rosemary threaded on to a cocktail stick if desired.

SHAKE IT UP

OREO MILKSHAKE

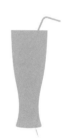

INGREDIENTS

200 ml milk
2 scoops chocolate ice cream
6 Oreo biscuits
Squirty cream, an extra Oreo cookie
   and chocolate sauce, to serve

METHOD

Place the milk and Oreo cookies into a blender and blend well. Add the chocolate ice cream and blend again until all the ingredients are combined. Pour into a tall glass (an old-fashioned sundae glass would really fit the bill) and if you want to go all out, top with squirty cream, Oreo biscuit crumbs and chocolate sauce. Dairy-free milk and ice cream are available, if required.

CLASSIC VANILLA MILKSHAKE

INGREDIENTS

200 ml milk
2 scoops vanilla ice cream
1 tsp vanilla extract
Squirty cream and chocolate sprinkles,
   to serve

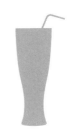

METHOD

Mix the ice cream, milk and vanilla extract in a blender until well combined. Pour into a tall glass or sundae glass and top with squirty cream and chocolate sprinkles. Use dairy-free milk and ice cream, if required.

STRAWBERRY PAVLOVA MILKSHAKE

INGREDIENTS

200 ml strawberry milk
2 scoops vanilla ice cream
8 strawberries
Squirty cream, strawberries and
    2–3 mini-meringues, to serve

METHOD

Add the strawberry milk, ice cream and strawberries to a blender and mix well until combined. Pour into a tall glass or sundae glass and top with squirty cream, more strawberries if desired and the mini-meringues. You might need to serve this one with a spoon! Opt for dairy-free milk and ice cream, if required.

TIP *If you really want to get into the baby-themed swing of things, you might want to serve your mocktails in baby bottles. This is likely to work best with the non-fizzy, less gloopy recipes in this section.*

PARTY SNACKS

THE FRIDGE IS A CLEAR EXAMPLE THAT WHAT MATTERS IS ON THE INSIDE.

★ *Anonymous* ★

As well as some finger foods suitable for any style of party, it might be fun to pepper in a few geared towards the impending arrival.

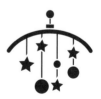

MAC AND CHEESE TOTS

INGREDIENTS (MAKES 30)

225 g mature cheddar cheese, grated

200 ml full-fat milk

125 g macaroni

30 g cream cheese (pasteurised)

20 g butter

20 g plain flour

1 egg

Salt and pepper, to taste

METHOD

Cook the macaroni according to instructions on the packet, drain and place to one side. Preheat the oven to 200°C. Take two mini-muffin tins and grease with oil. Add the butter and flour to a saucepan and whisk over a medium heat. Add the milk bit by bit, stirring every now and again until the mixture thickens and coats the back of a wooden spoon. Add the cream cheese and 200 g of the grated cheddar. Add salt and pepper to taste and stir all ingredients until smooth. Remove from heat and allow to cool for 5 minutes. Beat the egg and add it to the cheesy mixture, along with the macaroni. Spoon the mixture into the muffin tins and add a little of the remaining grated cheese to each one. Add further salt and pepper if you wish. Bake until the bites are golden brown – around 15–20 minutes – remove from oven and flip each bite over to cook the other side. Return to oven for a further 10 minutes. These can be served hot or cold.

PIGS IN BLANKETS

INGREDIENTS

Chipolatas (use twice as many as you have guests attending)

Rashers of smoked, streaky bacon (one for each chipolata)

3 tbsp Worcestershire sauce

1 tsp agave syrup

METHOD

Preheat the oven to 180°C. Take a rasher of bacon and lay it on a chopping board. Place a chipolata at one end, then roll it up in the bacon and place on a baking tray. When all pigs are firmly ensconced in their blankets, pop them in the oven for 30 minutes or until nice and crispy. Remove from oven, and drizzle over the Worcestershire sauce and agave syrup, give the baking tray a good shake to coat the pigs nicely and pop back in the oven for 2 minutes. Serve with a little pot of ketchup and one of mustard for dipping.

READY-TO-POP POPCORN

INGREDIENTS (MAKES A LARGE BOWL)

100 g popcorn kernels
3 tsp coconut oil
1 tbsp butter, melted (optional)
Salt, to taste

METHOD

Heat the coconut oil in a large pan (to test if the pan is hot enough, place a couple of kernels in the pan to see if they pop) and add the kernels. Place the lid on the saucepan and remove from the heat for 30 seconds. Return to the heat, giving the pan a gentle shake every now and then until the popping slows. When the pops have stopped, remove from heat and voila. If you want to make them extra-indulgent, drizzle over the melted butter to taste and shake the pan. Add salt to taste and sprinkle with a little cinnamon if desired. Other ideas for toppings: sugar, desiccated coconut, honey, paprika, curry powder or grated Parmesan.

MINI-BLT BONNETS

INGREDIENTS

5–6 strips of streaky bacon

Jar of mayonnaise

Chipotle sauce

24 cherry tomatoes

1 round lettuce (you could use spinach, rocket or other
  greens, if you prefer)

METHOD

Cook the bacon until crispy and leave to cool. Crumble 3–4 strips into a bowl and set to one side. Chop the rest of the bacon into pieces of about 1 cm width. In another bowl, mix the mayonnaise with chipotle sauce to taste. You could use paprika or chilli powder if there is no chipotle sauce to hand. Set this to one side. Now take the tomatoes and cut off the bottom bit (i.e. not the bit where the stalk once was as this will form its base). Remove the tomatoes' 'innards' so you're just left with the shells. Place a small piece of greens into each tomato shell and add a large pinch (around ½ tsp) of the crumbled bacon on top. Then add a small dollop of the mayo (you might want to pipe this through a piping bag/plastic sandwich bag with the corner cut for ease) and pop one of the bacon pieces on top. Voila!

PIZZA PRAM WHEELS

INGREDIENTS

For the pastry (you can buy ready-made pastry if pushed for time):
250 g self-raising flour
150 g milk
50 g margarine

For the toppings:
200 g tomato purée
100 g grated mozzarella (pasteurised)
50g grated cheddar
1 tsp dried oregano
1 tsp dried basil
Other toppings of your choice: salami, pepperoni, red onion, tuna, chicken, peppers, sweetcorn, etc.

METHOD

Preheat oven to 220°C. Sieve the flour into a mixing bowl and rub in the margarine until the mixture looks like breadcrumbs. Add the milk and combine to a soft dough. Dust a surface with flour, transfer the dough and knead gently. Using a rolling pin, roll the dough out to roughly the size of an A4 piece of paper. Spread tomato purée over the pastry, sprinkle cheese, herbs and any other toppings and carefully roll up the dough into a long tube. Slice into 8–10 pieces and place on a baking tray. Dab the pinwheels with a little oil (if you have a spray dispenser of oil, even better) and bake for 10–15 minutes until golden.

STUFFED SWEET POTATO SKINS

INGREDIENTS (MAKES 8)

4 sweet potatoes

100 g mozzarella, grated

100 g cheddar, grated

60 ml milk

1 tbsp olive oil

4 strips streaky bacon

Salt and pepper, to taste

Sour cream and chives, chopped, to serve

METHOD

Preheat the oven to 200°C. Pierce the sweet potatoes a few times with a fork and place on a baking tray. Cook for 50 minutes and leave to cool. Once cooled, cut potatoes in half lengthways and scoop out the flesh, leaving only a thin layer of potato inside, and place the flesh in a bowl. Return the potato skins to baking tray, drizzle with olive oil and bake for 10 minutes. Add the milk, salt and pepper to the potato flesh and mix well. Fill the potato skins with the mixture. Mix the two cheeses together in a bowl and top the potato skins with a generous amount. Bake these at 200°C for 15 minutes. While these are cooking, grill the bacon until crispy and crumble into a bowl. Once the cheese has melted on the potato skins, remove from oven and top with bacon bits. Serve with sour cream topped with chopped chives.

FRUIT TRAY PRAM

INGREDIENTS

1 large watermelon
1 orange
4 glacé cherries
1 pineapple
1 block mild cheddar cheese
cocktail sticks

For the fruit filling
(you can adapt this to your tastes):
2 punnets blueberries
2 punnets strawberries

METHOD

To turn the watermelon into a pram shape, slice out one-quarter of the melon by positioning a sharp, hefty knife on top of the fruit and cutting into it until the knife is about halfway through the melon. Turn the watermelon 90°, and cut into it a second time to meet the first cut, and remove the wedge – so a quarter of the watermelon should have been removed. Carefully hollow out the melon shell from the remaining three-quarters and cut the removed watermelon flesh into chunks. Place the melon shell on to a platter so the gap is at the front and it looks like a baby's pram. Arrange some of the chopped watermelon flesh at its base. Slice the orange and, using cocktail sticks, attach one slice to each 'corner' of the bottom of the melon shell, popping a glacé cherry on the end of each cocktail stick, creating the pram's wheels. Skewer chunks of pineapple and cheese on the cocktail sticks and arrange around the base of the melon. Then fill the 'pram' with blueberries, strawberries and the rest of the watermelon – and indeed any other fruits you would like to include. This makes a great centrepiece to a baby shower buffet table.

NO-BAKE BABY CHEESECAKES

INGREDIENTS

250 ml double cream
225 g cream cheese
100 g caster sugar
85 g digestive biscuits
25 g unsalted butter
2 tsp lemon zest
1 tsp vanilla extract
Dark chocolate, flaked
Strawberries, sliced

METHOD

Place the digestive biscuits into a plastic sandwich bag, seal and bash with a rolling pin until reduced to crumbs (alternatively, you can use a food processer, but where's the fun in that?). Transfer to a large bowl. Melt the butter in a pan or the microwave and place into the bowl with the biscuit crumbs; mix well. Set out as many ramekins as you have guests, and place 2 tbsp into each and press down. In another bowl, whisk together the cream cheese and sugar. Stir in the vanilla extract and lemon zest and set to one side. Take another bowl and whisk the cream into peaks. Bit by bit, gently fold the cream into the cream cheese and sugar mixture. Spoon into each serving vessel, leaving a little room at the top for the fruit. Chop the strawberries however you like and add a small handful to the top of each mini-cheesecake. Sprinkle with chocolate flakes as desired.

CAKES, CAKES, CAKES

A cake is often the centrepiece of a baby shower – whether it's in the shape of a pram or some other piece of baby paraphernalia, or if you're feeling extra brave on the creative front: an actual baby – and some choose to use it to do a dramatic gender reveal. A little old-fashioned, perhaps, but some mothers-to-be like to opt for either blue or pink icing on their baby shower cake to reveal to the other guests whether they are having a baby boy or a girl. Others prefer the words 'It's a boy!' or 'It's a girl', in any colour of their choosing, which would work just as well. Make sure you have your best baker on hand to knock up something special, or if your guests are devoid of time or baking talent, then order one in advance so it can be personalised.

RESOURCES

GOOD ORDER IS THE FOUNDATION OF ALL THINGS.

★ *Edmund Burke* ★

ACTIVITIES A–Z

Canal boat trip: www.narrowboats.org

Chocolate-making: www.mychocolate.co.uk

Greyhound racing: www.gbgb.org.uk

Horse racing: www.britishhorseracing.com

Jewellery-making: www.handmadehen.co.uk

Karaoke: www.luckyvoice.com,
www.brazenmonkey.co.uk, www.karaokebox.co.uk

Perfume-making: www.theperfumestudio.com

Pubs: www.thegoodpubguide.co.uk

RSPB nature reserves: www.rspb.org.uk

Soap-making: www.littlesoapcompany.co.uk

Spas: www.groupon.co.uk, www.livingsocial.co.uk,
www.spabreaks.com, www.spaseekers.com

Theatre tickets: www.ticketmaster.co.uk

Vintage-themed tea parties/makeovers:
www.hopeandgloriousvintage.blogspot.com,
www.teaandtrim.com

Walking: www.nationaltrail.co.uk,
www.walkengland.org.uk

Wildfowl & Wetlands Trust: www.wwt.org.uk

ACCOMMODATION

Boats: www.waterwaysholidays.com, www.drifters.co.uk

Campsites: www.coolcamping.co.uk

Center Parcs: www.centerparcs.co.uk

Forest cabins: www.forestholidays.co.uk

Group accommodation: www.homeaway.co.uk, www.groupaccommodation.com, www.airbnb.com, www.bigholidayhouse.com

Hotels/B&Bs: www.hotels.com, www.trivago.co.uk

Youth hostels: www.yha.org.uk

HEN
PARTY

planning

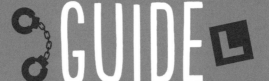

GUIDE

Verity Davidson